Beyond Boundaries: A Journey into the Science and Art of Extending Lifespan

"Exploring the Frontiers of Human Longevity and Well-being"

Clara Greene

Table of contents

Introduction
Chapter 1
Chapter 2
Chapter 3
Chapter 4
Chapter 5
Chapter 6
Chapter 7
Chapter 8
Chapter 9

Introduction

Welcome to "Beyond Boundaries: A Journey into the Science and Art of Extending Lifespan," a comprehensive exploration into the fascinating realm of extending human lifespan and improving healthspan. In this introductory chapter, we embark on a journey to understand the essence of life extension, its significance in our lives, and the overarching themes that guide our exploration.

The Quest for Longevity: Defining Life Extension

Life extension, once relegated to the realms of science fiction and myth, has emerged as a tangible and burgeoning field of scientific inquiry. At its core, life extension encompasses the pursuit of extending human lifespan beyond its natural limits while enhancing the quality of life during those additional years. It delves into the intricate mechanisms of aging, seeking to unravel its mysteries and unlock the secrets to prolonged vitality.

Understanding Aging: A Complex Tapestry

Central to the concept of life extension is the understanding of aging itself. Aging is a multifaceted process, influenced by an interplay of genetic, environmental, and lifestyle factors. It manifests at various levels, from the molecular intricacies within our cells to the physiological changes observable in our bodies over time. By comprehending the mechanisms driving aging, we gain insight into how to potentially intervene and mitigate its effects.

The Significance of Life Extension

The quest for life extension holds profound significance in the fabric of human existence. It speaks to our innate desire for longevity, for the opportunity to experience more of the world, to accomplish our dreams, and to cherish moments with loved ones. Beyond individual aspirations, life extension carries broader societal implications, ranging from healthcare sustainability to economic productivity. By extending healthy lifespan, we pave the way for a brighter, more vibrant future for generations to come.

Purpose and Scope of the Book

"Beyond Boundaries" aims to be a definitive guide, synthesizing the latest scientific advancements, ethical considerations, and practical strategies in the realm of life extension. Our journey will traverse the landscape of aging research, from elucidating the biological mechanisms of aging to exploring cutting-edge interventions and contemplating the ethical dilemmas that accompany such endeavors.

Navigating the Chapters Ahead

As you delve into the chapters that follow, prepare to embark on a voyage of discovery. Each chapter is meticulously crafted to illuminate a different facet of life extension, offering insights, practical tips, and thought-provoking discussions. Whether you're a seasoned researcher, a curious enthusiast, or someone simply intrigued by the possibility of a longer, healthier life, "Beyond Boundaries" invites you to join the quest for extended vitality and enhanced well-being.

With anticipation and excitement, let us embark on this extraordinary journey together.

Chapter 1

Understanding Aging

In the intricate tapestry of life, aging stands as one of the most enigmatic and universally experienced phenomena. From the moment of our birth, we embark on a journey inexorably intertwined with the passage of time, marked by the gradual unfolding of aging processes within our bodies. In this chapter, we embark on a voyage of discovery to unravel the complexities of aging, delving deep into its biological underpinnings, exploring the theories that seek to explain its mechanisms, and contemplating its profound implications for human existence.

Biological Processes of Aging

At its essence, aging is a dynamic and multifaceted process that manifests across multiple levels of biological organization. From the molecular intricacies within our cells to the systemic changes observable in our bodies, aging leaves an indelible mark on every aspect of our being. Key hallmarks of aging include genomic instability, telomere attrition, epigenetic alterations, loss of proteostasis, mitochondrial dysfunction, cellular senescence, stem cell exhaustion, and altered intercellular communication. These interconnected processes converge to drive the progressive decline in physiological function that characterizes aging.

Theories of Aging

To comprehend aging fully, we must grapple with the diverse array of theories proposed to explain its underlying mechanisms. From the evolutionary perspective, aging is viewed as the result of evolutionary trade-offs that favor reproductive success over longevity. The mitochondrial theory of aging posits that accumulated damage to mitochondrial DNA leads to impaired energy production and increased oxidative stress, contributing to cellular dysfunction and aging. The free radical theory of aging implicates reactive oxygen species in the gradual deterioration of cellular structures and functions. Additionally, the telomere theory of aging highlights the role of telomere shortening in driving cellular senescence and age-related decline.

Genetic and Environmental Factors

Aging represents a complex interplay between genetic predispositions and environmental influences. While our genetic makeup lays the foundation for our susceptibility to age-related diseases and longevity, environmental factors such as diet, exercise, stress, exposure to toxins, and social interactions exert profound effects on the aging process. Epigenetic modifications, which regulate gene expression without altering the underlying DNA sequence, serve as a crucial interface between our genes and the environment, shaping our responses to external stimuli and influencing the trajectory of aging.

Implications for Life Extension

Understanding the intricacies of aging holds profound implications for the quest to extend human lifespan and improve healthspan. By elucidating the molecular and cellular mechanisms driving aging, researchers can identify potential targets for interventions aimed at slowing or reversing the aging process. From pharmacological interventions that target age-related pathways to lifestyle modifications that promote healthy aging, the insights gleaned from the study of aging offer hope for a future where age-related diseases are conquered, and individuals enjoy longer, healthier lives.

As we delve deeper into the mysteries of aging, let us remain ever mindful of the profound significance of our quest. For in our pursuit of extended vitality lies the promise of a future where the boundaries of human potential are transcended, and the joys of life are savored to their fullest extent.

Chapter 2

Extending Lifespan

In the quest to transcend the limitations of human mortality, the pursuit of extending lifespan stands as a paramount endeavor. This chapter delves into the scientific advancements, emerging technologies, and innovative strategies that hold the promise of prolonging human lifespan and enhancing the quality of life in our later years.

Cellular Mechanisms of Aging

Central to the quest for life extension is the elucidation of the intricate cellular mechanisms underlying aging. From the gradual accumulation of DNA damage to the dysregulation of cellular signaling pathways, aging unfolds as a complex interplay of molecular processes within our cells. Key targets for intervention include the mitigation of oxidative stress, the restoration of mitochondrial function, and the promotion of cellular repair and regeneration. By understanding these fundamental mechanisms, researchers aim to develop targeted interventions capable of slowing or reversing the aging process at its core.

Role of Genetics in Longevity

Genetics plays a pivotal role in shaping an individual's susceptibility to age-related diseases and determining their overall lifespan. Through the study of centenarians and other long-lived populations, researchers have identified genetic variants associated with exceptional longevity, offering insights into the genetic determinants of aging. These include genes involved in DNA repair, inflammation, metabolism, and cellular senescence. Advances in genomics and genetic engineering hold the promise of harnessing these genetic insights to develop personalized interventions tailored to individual genetic profiles, ultimately paving the way for customized approaches to life extension.

Emerging Technologies in Life Extension

The landscape of life extension is continually evolving, driven by rapid advances in biotechnology, regenerative medicine, and computational biology. From the development of senolytic drugs that selectively target senescent cells to the use of CRISPR gene editing to correct age-related mutations, a plethora of innovative technologies are reshaping our understanding of aging and opening new avenues for intervention. Nanotechnology offers the potential for targeted drug delivery and tissue repair, while artificial intelligence revolutionizes drug discovery and personalized medicine. As these technologies converge, they hold the promise of ushering in a new era of personalized, precision medicine aimed at extending lifespan and enhancing healthspan.

Ethical and Social Considerations

While the prospect of life extension brings hope for a future of extended vitality and well-being, it also raises profound ethical and social considerations. Questions surrounding equity and access to life-extending technologies, the potential exacerbation of existing socioeconomic disparities, and the ethical implications of manipulating the fundamental processes of life demand careful consideration. Additionally, the psychological impact of life extension, including existential questions surrounding the nature of identity and the meaning of life in an ageless society, poses significant challenges that must be addressed thoughtfully.

As we stand on the precipice of a new era in the history of humanity, the quest for life extension beckons us forward with the promise of a future where the boundaries of human potential are transcended, and the joys of life are savored to their fullest extent. By harnessing the power of science, technology, and human ingenuity, we embark on a journey to unlock the secrets of longevity and shape a future where age is but a number, and the possibilities are limitless.

Chapter 3

Healthspan vs. Lifespan

In the pursuit of a longer and more fulfilling life, it is essential to distinguish between lifespan, the total duration of an individual's life, and healthspan, the period of life spent in good health, free from the burden of disease and disability. This chapter delves into the intricate interplay between healthspan and lifespan, exploring strategies to optimize both and foster a future where not only do we live longer, but we also live better.

Defining Healthspan and Lifespan

Healthspan and lifespan represent two distinct yet interconnected dimensions of human longevity. Lifespan, often measured in years, quantifies the total duration of an individual's life from birth to death. Healthspan, on the other hand, reflects the period of life characterized by optimal physical, mental, and social well-being, devoid of chronic illness, disability, or functional decline. While extending lifespan remains a central objective of life extension research, enhancing healthspan holds equal importance, as it ensures that the additional years gained are lived with vitality and purpose.

Strategies to Improve Healthspan

Achieving a longer healthspan requires a multifaceted approach that addresses the diverse determinants of health and well-being. Nutrition plays a central role, with evidence suggesting that a diet rich in fruits, vegetables, whole grains, and lean proteins can promote longevity and reduce the risk of age-related diseases. Regular physical activity is equally crucial, with exercise conferring numerous benefits, including improved cardiovascular health, enhanced cognitive function, and reduced risk of chronic conditions such as diabetes and osteoporosis. Adequate sleep, stress management, social engagement, and cognitive stimulation also contribute to optimal healthspan, fostering resilience and vitality as we age.

The Interplay Between Healthspan and Lifespan

While extending lifespan holds inherent value, it is essential to recognize that the quality of those additional years is equally significant. A focus solely on prolonging lifespan without addressing the determinants of healthspan risks prolonging the burden of age-related diseases and disability, undermining the overall quality of life. Conversely, efforts to enhance healthspan can indirectly contribute to extending lifespan by reducing the incidence of age-related morbidity and mortality. By optimizing both healthspan and lifespan, individuals can enjoy not only a longer life but also a life filled with vitality, purpose, and meaning.

Challenges and Opportunities

Despite the growing recognition of the importance of healthspan, numerous challenges remain on the path to achieving optimal aging for all. Socioeconomic disparities, unequal access to healthcare, and environmental factors such as pollution and climate change pose significant barriers to healthspan optimization, disproportionately affecting vulnerable populations. Addressing these challenges requires a multifaceted approach that encompasses not only individual behavior change but also systemic interventions aimed at promoting health equity and social justice. By fostering a supportive environment that enables all individuals to live healthier, more fulfilling lives, we can work towards a future where healthspan is maximized, and the potential for human flourishing is realized.

As we navigate the complexities of aging in the 21st century, the distinction between healthspan and lifespan emerges as a guiding principle in our quest for extended vitality and well-being. By embracing strategies that optimize both dimensions of human longevity, we can forge a future where age is not a barrier but a celebration of a life lived to its fullest potential.

Chapter 4

Lifestyle Interventions

In the pursuit of longevity and well-being, lifestyle interventions stand as pillars of preventive medicine, offering powerful tools to promote healthspan and optimize the quality of life as we age. This chapter delves into the multifaceted landscape of lifestyle interventions, exploring the impact of nutrition, exercise, sleep, and other modifiable behaviors on human longevity and vitality.

Nutrition and Diet

Nutrition plays a pivotal role in shaping healthspan, influencing a myriad of biological processes that impact aging and disease risk. A diet rich in fruits, vegetables, whole grains, and lean proteins provides essential nutrients, antioxidants, and phytochemicals that promote cellular health and resilience. The Mediterranean diet, characterized by its emphasis on plant-based foods, healthy fats, and moderate alcohol consumption, has garnered particular attention for its association with reduced risk of chronic diseases and enhanced longevity. Additionally, caloric restriction and intermittent fasting have emerged as dietary strategies that may confer longevity benefits by modulating metabolic pathways, reducing inflammation, and promoting cellular repair mechanisms.

Exercise and Physical Activity

Regular physical activity is a cornerstone of healthy aging, exerting a multitude of beneficial effects on physical, mental, and cognitive well-being. Aerobic exercise, such as brisk walking, jogging, swimming, or cycling, improves cardiovascular health, enhances endurance, and reduces the risk of chronic conditions such as heart disease and diabetes. Strength training exercises, including weightlifting and resistance training, promote muscle mass, bone density, and functional independence, mitigating the age-related decline in musculoskeletal health. Additionally, mind-body practices such as yoga, tai chi, and qigong offer holistic benefits, fostering relaxation, stress reduction, and emotional well-being.

Sleep Optimization

Quality sleep is essential for overall health and vitality, serving as a cornerstone of optimal aging. Adequate sleep duration and quality are associated with a myriad of physiological processes, including hormone regulation, immune function, and cognitive performance. Chronic sleep deprivation, on the other hand, is linked to an increased risk of obesity, diabetes, cardiovascular disease, and cognitive decline. Strategies to optimize sleep include maintaining a consistent sleep schedule, creating a relaxing bedtime routine, optimizing sleep environment, and avoiding stimulants such as caffeine and electronics before bedtime. Addressing underlying sleep disorders such as sleep apnea and insomnia is also crucial for promoting restorative sleep and enhancing overall healthspan.

Stress Management and Mindfulness

Chronic stress exerts profound effects on physical and mental health, contributing to inflammation, oxidative stress, and dysregulation of stress hormones such as cortisol. Mind-body practices such as mindfulness meditation, deep breathing exercises, and progressive muscle relaxation offer powerful tools for stress reduction and emotional resilience. By cultivating present-moment awareness and fostering a sense of inner calm, mindfulness practices promote adaptive responses to stressors, enhance emotional regulation, and improve overall well-being.

In the tapestry of human longevity, lifestyle interventions stand as potent allies in the quest for extended vitality and well-being. By embracing a holistic approach to health that encompasses nutrition, exercise, sleep, stress management, and other modifiable behaviors, individuals can empower themselves to optimize their healthspan and savor the joys of life to their fullest extent.

Chapter 5

Medical Interventions

In the ongoing quest to extend human lifespan and enhance healthspan, medical interventions play a pivotal role, offering a spectrum of innovative approaches to mitigate age-related decline, prevent chronic diseases, and promote optimal aging. This chapter delves into the diverse array of medical interventions, from pharmacological therapies to regenerative medicine techniques, that hold the potential to revolutionize the landscape of human longevity and well-being.

Pharmacological Interventions

Pharmacological interventions represent one of the cornerstones of modern medicine's arsenal against age-related diseases and functional decline. From cardiovascular medications that lower blood pressure and cholesterol levels to antidiabetic drugs that improve glucose regulation and insulin sensitivity, pharmacotherapy targets a wide range of physiological pathways implicated in aging and disease. Additionally, novel therapeutics such as senolytics, which selectively target and eliminate senescent cells, hold promise for mitigating age-related inflammation and tissue dysfunction. Other emerging pharmacological interventions include metformin, rapamycin, and NAD+ precursors, which have been shown to extend lifespan and improve healthspan in preclinical studies and clinical trials.

Hormone Replacement Therapy

Hormone replacement therapy (HRT) offers another avenue for intervention in age-related hormonal imbalances that contribute to the deterioration of physiological function. In men, testosterone replacement therapy can alleviate symptoms of hypogonadism, including reduced libido, fatigue, and loss of muscle mass, while also potentially reducing the risk of cardiovascular disease and osteoporosis. Similarly, estrogen replacement therapy in postmenopausal women has been shown to alleviate menopausal symptoms, preserve bone density, and reduce the risk of cardiovascular events. However, the use of HRT is not without risks, and careful consideration of individual risk factors and potential side effects is essential in clinical decision-making.

Stem Cell Therapy

Regenerative medicine approaches, such as stem cell therapy, offer novel strategies for repairing and rejuvenating aging tissues and organs. Stem cells possess the unique ability to differentiate into various cell types and promote tissue regeneration, making them promising candidates for treating age-related degenerative conditions such as osteoarthritis, neurodegenerative diseases, and cardiovascular disorders. Mesenchymal stem cells, derived from sources such as bone marrow, adipose tissue, and umbilical cord blood, have shown therapeutic potential in preclinical and clinical studies for their ability to modulate inflammation, promote tissue repair, and enhance functional recovery. Additionally, induced pluripotent stem cells (iPSCs) hold promise for personalized regenerative therapies by enabling the generation of patient-specific cells for transplantation and disease modeling.

Challenges and Considerations

Despite the promise of medical interventions in extending lifespan and enhancing healthspan, several challenges and considerations must be addressed. These include safety concerns associated with pharmacological therapies, ethical considerations surrounding the use of stem cells and genetic interventions, and regulatory hurdles in translating promising preclinical findings into clinical applications. Additionally, the cost and accessibility of medical interventions may pose barriers to equitable access, underscoring the importance of addressing health disparities and ensuring that life-extending technologies are available to all.

As we navigate the frontiers of medical science and technology, the promise of medical interventions in extending human lifespan and promoting optimal aging shines bright. By harnessing the power of pharmacotherapy, hormone replacement therapy, stem cell therapy, and other innovative approaches, we pave the way for a future where age-related diseases are conquered, and individuals enjoy longer, healthier lives filled with vitality and purpose.

Chapter 6

Cutting-edge Research

In the relentless pursuit of extending human lifespan and enhancing healthspan, cutting-edge research serves as the vanguard, pushing the boundaries of scientific knowledge and technological innovation to unlock the secrets of aging and rejuvenation. This chapter delves into the forefront of aging research, exploring the latest discoveries, breakthrough technologies, and promising interventions that hold the potential to reshape the landscape of human longevity and well-being.

CRISPR Technology and Gene Editing

CRISPR-Cas9 technology has emerged as a revolutionary tool in the field of genetics, offering unprecedented precision and versatility in genome editing. By harnessing the power of CRISPR, researchers can precisely modify DNA sequences, correct disease-causing mutations, and engineer novel genetic constructs with unparalleled efficiency. In the realm of aging research, CRISPR holds promise for elucidating the genetic basis of longevity, identifying therapeutic targets for age-related diseases, and exploring innovative approaches to rejuvenation. Applications of CRISPR technology in aging research include the manipulation of key genes involved in cellular senescence, DNA repair, and metabolic regulation, paving the way for targeted interventions to promote healthy aging and extend lifespan.

Senolytics and Senescence

Cellular senescence, the irreversible arrest of cell proliferation accompanied by a pro-inflammatory phenotype, plays a central role in aging and age-related diseases. Senolytics are a class of drugs that selectively target and eliminate senescent cells, thereby attenuating age-related inflammation, tissue dysfunction, and functional decline. By clearing senescent cells, senolytics hold promise for rejuvenating aging tissues, delaying the onset of age-related pathologies, and extending healthspan. Ongoing research efforts focus on identifying novel senolytic compounds, optimizing drug delivery methods, and elucidating the molecular mechanisms underlying senescence and senolytic action.

Telomere Lengthening

Telomeres, the protective caps at the ends of chromosomes, play a crucial role in maintaining genomic stability and cellular function. Telomere shortening, a hallmark of aging, is associated with cellular senescence, genomic instability, and increased susceptibility to age-related diseases. Strategies to lengthen telomeres hold promise for reversing age-related telomere attrition, promoting cellular rejuvenation, and extending lifespan. Telomerase activation, telomere-targeting gene therapies, and telomere elongation through lifestyle interventions represent promising avenues for telomere lengthening research. Additionally, emerging technologies such as telomere extension by synthetic oligonucleotides (TESO) offer innovative approaches to telomere length modulation and age reversal.

Ethical and Regulatory Considerations

As research in aging and longevity advances, it is essential to address the ethical, social, and regulatory implications of emerging technologies and interventions. Ethical considerations include questions surrounding equitable access to life-extending treatments, the potential exacerbation of existing health disparities, and the ethical use of genetic interventions to enhance human lifespan. Regulatory challenges encompass the need for robust oversight of emerging technologies, ensuring safety, efficacy, and equitable distribution of life-extending interventions. Additionally, societal attitudes towards aging, longevity, and the pursuit of immortality shape the discourse surrounding cutting-edge research in aging, highlighting the importance of fostering informed public dialogue and ethical reflection.

As we stand at the precipice of a new era in the study of aging and longevity, the possibilities are boundless. Through the convergence of cutting-edge research, transformative technologies, and collaborative efforts across disciplines, we hold the keys to unlocking the secrets of aging and reshaping the trajectory of human lifespan and well-being. With unwavering dedication, scientific ingenuity, and ethical foresight, we embark on a journey towards a future where age is but a number, and the potential for human flourishing knows no bounds.

Chapter 7

Ethical and Social Implications

In the pursuit of extending human lifespan and enhancing healthspan, ethical and social considerations loom large, shaping the discourse surrounding the implications of life-extending technologies and interventions. This chapter delves into the complex web of ethical dilemmas, social challenges, and moral imperatives that accompany the quest for longevity and well-being, inviting reflection and dialogue on the ethical and societal dimensions of life extension.

Equity and Access

One of the most pressing ethical considerations in the field of life extension revolves around equity and access to life-extending technologies and interventions. As life-extending therapies and interventions become available, questions arise regarding their distribution and affordability. Will life-extending treatments be accessible only to the wealthy elite, widening existing health disparities and exacerbating social inequality? Or will efforts be made to ensure equitable access, prioritizing the needs of marginalized and underserved populations? Addressing these questions requires a commitment to social justice and health equity, fostering policies and practices that promote fair and inclusive access to life-extending interventions for all.

Psychological Impact

The pursuit of longevity and the prospect of extended lifespan raise profound psychological implications for individuals and society as a whole. Existential questions surrounding the nature of identity, the meaning of life, and the inevitability of death come to the forefront, challenging deeply held beliefs and cultural norms. Fear of aging and mortality may give rise to anxiety, depression, and existential distress, while the pursuit of eternal youth may fuel narcissism, hedonism, and a disregard for the value of human life. Additionally, societal attitudes towards aging and longevity shape perceptions of worth, dignity, and societal contribution, influencing individual choices and societal priorities.

Ethical Use of Technology

Advances in biotechnology, genetics, and regenerative medicine offer unprecedented opportunities to manipulate the fundamental processes of life and reshape the trajectory of human aging. However, with these advances come ethical considerations regarding the responsible use of technology and the potential consequences of genetic enhancement and manipulation. Questions arise regarding the ethical implications of gene editing, stem cell therapy, and other interventions aimed at extending lifespan and enhancing human capabilities. What are the potential risks and unintended consequences of genetic interventions? How do we ensure the autonomy, dignity, and well-being of individuals in the pursuit of life extension? These questions demand careful consideration and ethical reflection, guiding responsible innovation and decision-making in the realm of life extension research and practice.

Cultural and Societal Attitudes

Cultural and societal attitudes towards aging, longevity, and the pursuit of life extension vary widely across different cultures and societies, reflecting diverse values, beliefs, and worldviews. In some cultures, aging is revered as a natural and inevitable part of the life cycle, while in others, youthfulness and vitality are prized above all else. Attitudes towards death and dying also shape perceptions of life extension, with some embracing the inevitability of mortality as an essential aspect of the human experience, while others seek to defy death at all costs. Understanding and respecting cultural and societal diversity is essential in navigating the ethical and social complexities of life extension, fostering dialogue and collaboration across cultural boundaries.

As we navigate the ethical and social implications of life extension, we are called to engage in thoughtful reflection, dialogue, and action. By addressing issues of equity and access, grappling with existential questions, upholding ethical principles, and respecting cultural diversity, we can navigate the complexities of life extension with wisdom, compassion, and integrity. Ultimately, our collective efforts to promote human flourishing and well-being must be guided by a commitment to justice, equity, and the common good, ensuring that the benefits of life extension are shared by all members of society.

Chapter 8

Future Perspectives

As we peer into the horizon of human longevity and well-being, the future holds boundless possibilities, ripe with promise and potential. This chapter offers a visionary exploration of the future of life extension, contemplating emerging trends, transformative technologies, and paradigm shifts that may shape the trajectory of human aging and vitality in the years to come.

Potential Breakthroughs in Life Extension

The future of life extension is propelled by a wave of scientific discovery, technological innovation, and interdisciplinary collaboration, paving the way for unprecedented breakthroughs in our understanding of aging and rejuvenation. From the elucidation of novel aging pathways to the development of targeted interventions and personalized therapies, the pace of progress in aging research shows no signs of slowing. Emerging fields such as geroscience, systems biology, and artificial intelligence offer new insights and approaches to unraveling the complexities of aging, driving the development of innovative strategies to extend healthspan and lifespan.

Challenges and Barriers

Despite the promise of progress, the journey towards extended vitality and well-being is not without its challenges and barriers. Socioeconomic disparities, inadequate access to healthcare, regulatory hurdles, and ethical dilemmas pose significant obstacles to the equitable distribution and implementation of life-extending interventions. Additionally, societal attitudes towards aging, longevity, and the pursuit of immortality shape public discourse and policy priorities, influencing the direction of research and the allocation of resources. Addressing these challenges requires a multifaceted approach that encompasses scientific innovation, policy reform, and social advocacy, fostering a supportive environment for the advancement of aging research and turning scientific breakthroughs into practical advantages for the community.

The Future of Aging Research

Looking ahead, the future of aging research holds immense promise for transformative breakthroughs that may revolutionize the field and reshape our understanding of human aging and longevity. From the development of precision medicine approaches tailored to individual genetic profiles to the exploration of novel interventions targeting the hallmarks of aging, researchers are poised to unlock new frontiers in the quest for extended vitality and well-being. Emerging technologies such as gene editing, stem cell therapy, and regenerative medicine offer unprecedented opportunities to intervene in the aging process at its root, paving the way for a future where age-related diseases are conquered, and individuals enjoy longer, healthier lives free from the burden of chronic illness and disability.

Shaping the Future Together

As we stand on the threshold of a new era in the history of humanity, the future of life extension beckons us forward with the promise of a world where age is but a number, and the possibilities for human flourishing are limitless. By embracing a collective vision of extended vitality, fostering interdisciplinary collaboration, and championing ethical principles and social justice, we can shape a future where the joys of life are savored to their fullest extent, and the potential for human achievement knows no bounds.

As we gaze into the horizon of human longevity and well-being, let us do so with hope, determination, and unwavering optimism. The future of life extension holds the promise of a world where age is no longer a barrier but a celebration of the resilience, wisdom, and vitality of the human spirit. By harnessing the power of science, technology, and human ingenuity, we embark on a journey towards a future where every individual has the opportunity to outlive, thrive, and flourish in a world filled with endless possibilities.

Chapter 9

Conclusion

As we draw the curtains on our exploration of the science and art of life extension, we reflect on the journey we have undertaken, the discoveries we have made, and the possibilities that lie ahead. This concluding chapter offers a moment of reflection, a celebration of our collective quest for extended vitality and well-being, and a call to action for the future.

A Journey of Discovery

Our journey began with a deep dive into the intricacies of aging, unraveling the mysteries of cellular senescence, genetic determinants of longevity, and the interconnected pathways that shape our aging trajectory. From there, we explored the diverse array of lifestyle interventions, medical therapies, and cutting-edge research that hold the promise of extending human lifespan and enhancing healthspan. Along the way, we grappled with ethical dilemmas, social implications, and existential questions, navigating the complexities of life extension with wisdom, compassion, and foresight.

The Promise of Possibility

As we stand at the crossroads of human longevity, the future brims with possibility and promise. Advances in biotechnology, regenerative medicine, and artificial intelligence offer unprecedented opportunities to intervene in the aging process, reshape the trajectory of human lifespan, and promote optimal aging for all. From the development of personalized therapies tailored to individual genetic profiles to the exploration of novel interventions targeting the fundamental hallmarks of aging, the pace of progress in aging research shows no signs of slowing. With each new discovery, each breakthrough innovation, we inch closer towards a future where age-related diseases are conquered, and individuals enjoy longer, healthier lives filled with vitality and purpose.

A Call to Action

As we contemplate the future of life extension, we are called to action. The quest for extended vitality and well-being is not the pursuit of a select few but a collective endeavor that demands the engagement and collaboration of individuals, communities, and societies worldwide. We must advocate for policies and practices that promote health equity and social justice, ensuring that life-extending interventions are accessible to all members of society. We must foster interdisciplinary collaboration and scientific innovation, driving the development of transformative technologies and interventions that address the root causes of aging and disease. And above all, we must embrace a vision of aging that celebrates the resilience, wisdom, and diversity of the human experience, recognizing that age is not a barrier but a celebration of life's journey.

Embracing the Journey Ahead

As we bid farewell to the pages of this book, let us carry forth the lessons learned, the insights gained, and the dreams that fuel our quest for extended vitality and well-being. The journey of life extension is not a destination but a continuous evolution, a journey of discovery, growth, and transformation that unfolds with each passing day. With curiosity as our compass, resilience as our guide, and compassion as our North Star, let us embrace the journey ahead with open hearts and open minds, knowing that together, we have the power to shape a future where every individual has the opportunity to outlive, thrive, and flourish in a world filled with endless possibilities.

Finally, we extend our heartfelt gratitude to all who have joined us on this journey—the researchers, scientists, innovators, and visionaries who illuminate the path forward, and the readers, enthusiasts, and advocates who fuel our collective quest for extended vitality and well-being. Together, we embark on a journey towards a future where age is not a barrier but a celebration of life's journey, and the potential for human flourishing knows no bounds.

With anticipation and gratitude, let us embrace the journey ahead.

www.ingramcontent.com/pod-product-compliance
Lightning Source LLC
Chambersburg PA
CBHW051854250726
48659CB00006B/2194